HOW THE LACK OF HIGHER EDUCATION FACULTY CONTRIBUTES TO AMERICA'S NURSING SHORTAGE, PART I

FIELD HEARING

BEFORE THE

SUBCOMMITTEE ON SELECT EDUCATION

OF THE

COMMITTEE ON EDUCATION AND THE WORKFORCE
U.S. HOUSE OF REPRESENTATIVES

ONE HUNDRED NINTH CONGRESS

FIRST SESSION

___

November 30, 2005 in Greeley, Colorado

___

Serial No. 109-29

___

Printed for the use of the Committee on Education and the Workforce

___

Available via the World Wide Web: http://www.access.gpo.gov/congress/house

or

Committee address: http://edworkforce.house.gov

___

U.S. GOVERNMENT PRINTING OFFICE

25-552 PDF   WASHINGTON : 2006

___

COMMITTEE ON EDUCATION AND THE WORKFORCE

JOHN A. BOEHNER, Ohio, *Chairman*

Thomas E. Petri, Wisconsin, *Vice Chairman*
Howard P. "Buck" McKeon, California
Michael N. Castle, Delaware
Sam Johnson, Texas
Mark E. Souder, Indiana
Charlie Norwood, Georgia
Vernon J. Ehlers, Michigan
Judy Biggert, Illinois
Todd Russell Platts, Pennsylvania
Patrick J. Tiberi, Ohio
Ric Keller, Florida
Tom Osborne, Nebraska
Joe Wilson, South Carolina
Jon C. Porter, Nevada
John Kline, Minnesota
Marilyn N. Musgrave, Colorado
Bob Inglis, South Carolina
Cathy McMorris, Washington
Kenny Marchant, Texas
Tom Price, Georgia
Luis G. Fortuño, Puerto Rico
Bobby Jindal, Louisiana
Charles W. Boustany, Jr., Louisiana
Virginia Foxx, North Carolina
Thelma D. Drake, Virginia
John R. "Randy" Kuhl, Jr., New York

George Miller, California
Dale E. Kildee, Michigan
Major R. Owens, New York
Donald M. Payne, New Jersey
Robert E. Andrews, New Jersey
Robert C. Scott, Virginia
Lynn C. Woolsey, California
Rubén Hinojosa, Texas
Carolyn McCarthy, New York
John F. Tierney, Massachusetts
Ron Kind, Wisconsin
Dennis J. Kucinich, Ohio
David Wu, Oregon
Rush D. Holt, New Jersey
Susan A. Davis, California
Betty McCollum, Minnesota
Danny K. Davis, Illinois
Raúl M. Grijalva, Arizona
Chris Van Hollen, Maryland
Tim Ryan, Ohio
Timothy H. Bishop, New York
John Barrow, Georgia

Paula Nowakowski, *Staff Director*
Mark Zuckerman, *Minority Staff Director*

SUBCOMMITTEE ON SELECT EDUCATION

PATRICK J. TIBERI, Ohio, *Chairman*

Cathy McMorris, Washington *Vice Chairman*
Mark E. Souder, Indiana
Jon C. Porter, Nevada
Bob Inglis, South Carolina
Luis P. Fortuño, Puerto Rico
John A. Boehner, Ohio, *ex officio*

Rubén Hinojosa, Texas
Danny K. Davis, Illinois
Chris Van Hollen, Maryland
Tim Ryan, Ohio
George Miller, California, *ex officio*

C O N T E N T S

HOW THE LACK OF HIGHER EDUCATION FAC-
ULTY CONTRIBUTES TO AMERICA'S NURS-
ING SHORTAGE, PART I

Thursday, November 30, 2005
U.S. House of Representatives
Subcommittee on Select Education
Committee on Education and the Workforce
Greeley, Colorado

The Subcommittee met, pursuant to call, at 10 a.m., at the University of Northern Colorado, University Center, Panorama Room, 2045 10th Avenue, Greeley, Colorado, Hon. Marilyn Musgrave presiding.

Present: Representatives Musgrave and Porter.

Mrs. MUSGRAVE. A quorum being present, the Subcommittee on Select Education of the Committee on Education in the Workforce will come to order.

We are meeting today to hear testimony on how the lack of higher education faculty contributes to America's nursing shortage.

I am very pleased to be here in Greeley today, and I'm eager to hear from our witnesses. But, before I begin, I ask for unanimous consent for the hearing to remain open for 14 days to allow Member statements and other extraneous material referred to during the hearing to be submitted in the official hearing record. Without objection, so ordered.

STATEMENT OF HON. MARILYN N. MUSGRAVE, A REPRESENTATIVE IN CONGRESS FROM THE STATE OF COLORADO

Mrs. MUSGRAVE. I'd like to thank all of you for being here today, and I certainly would like to extend my appreciation to Congressman Jon Porter for traveling to Greeley, and I do apologize for the weather, Congressman. It's a bit brutal today.

Mr. PORTER. It's a beautiful day.

Mrs. MUSGRAVE. And I'm glad that he's here to learn much about this urgent matter. He has been a leader on this issue, and I'm very grateful for the insight that he has.

We all know that our country is facing a nursing shortage that will have a significant impact on healthcare in our country. Last year, the U.S. Bureau of Labor Statistics projected that more than one million new and replacement nurses will be needed by 2012.

According to a 2002 health report, 44 states are expected to have shortages of registered nurses by the year 2020. In Colorado, the lack of registered nurses is twice the national average. The nursing shortage in our state is currently estimated to be 11 percent short of demand, and is expected to nearly triple to 30 percent by 2020 if current trends continue. This is a growing problem that demands our urgent attention.

Demand for nurses is projected to increase as population grows, baby boomers enter retirement, and medical advances extend our lifespans. In contrast, the supply of nursing professionals is expected to decline, as the number of nurses leaving the profession exceeds the number that are entering.

What many Americans do not realize is that this shortage is not simply a matter of inadequate enrollment in nursing schools. Thousands of qualified applicants to graduate nursing programs are turned away each year because there is a shortage of graduate-level nursing faculty.

A report by the American Association of Colleges of Nursing shows that U.S. Nursing schools turned away 32,797 qualified applicants from baccalaureate and graduate nursing programs in 2004 due to insignificant number of faculty, clinical sites, classroom space, and budget constraints. More than 2,600 applicants were turned away from the nursing program in Colorado—from nursing programs in Colorado, in 2003.

Three quarters of the nursing schools point to faculty shortages as a reason for not accepting all qualified applicants into nursing programs. This academic year, 66 percent of nursing schools report that they have vacancies and they are in need of additional nursing faculty to meet additional demand.

Colorado's shortage of qualified nursing faculty at its 2 year nursing schools is three times the national average, and nearly double the national average at its 4 year schools.

We anticipate this faculty shortage to escalate in the next decade due to budget constraints, increased job competition from clinics sites, and the retirement of a greying professional of the nursing faculty.

A wave of faculty retirements is expected within the next 10 years, between 200 and 300 doctrinally prepared faculty will be eligible for retirement each year from 2003 through 2012.

I am anxious to hear the testimony from our witnesses today. I very much appreciate your expertise and I'm proud of the efforts that are going on in Colorado to address the nursing shortage.

Colorado educational institutions and health care providers are working together to pursue strategies, to strengthen faculty recruitment and retention, and it's important for all of us that these efforts are very successful.

I hope that we can identify some strategies today that will address the problem of faculty shortage, and I also am very pleased to have Mr. Porter here, and I would now like to yield to him for any statements that he might have.

[The prepared statement of Mrs. Musgrave follows:]

Statement of Hon. Marilyn N. Musgrave, a Representative in Congress from the State of Colorado

Good morning. Thank you all for being here today. I would like to extend my appreciation to Congressman Jon Porter for traveling to Greeley to learn more about this urgent matter. He has been a leader on this issue and I am grateful for his insight this morning.

Our country is confronting a nursing shortage that will have a significant impact on the health care in our country. Last year, the U.S. Bureau of Labor Statistics projected that more than one million new and replacement nurses will be needed by 2012.

According to a 2002 health report, 44 states are expected to have shortages of registered nurses by the year 2020.

In Colorado, the lack of registered nurses is twice the national average. The nursing shortage in our state is currently estimated to be 11 percent short of demand, and is expected to nearly triple, to 30 percent, by 2020 if current trends continue. This is a growing problem that demands our urgent attention.

Demand for nurses is projected to increase as population grows, baby boomers enter retirement, and medical advances extend life span. In contrast, the supply of nursing professionals is expected to decline as the number of nurses leaving the profession exceeds the number that enter.

What many Americans do not realize is that this shortage is not simply a matter of inadequate enrollment in nursing programs. Thousands of qualified applicants to graduate nursing programs are turned away each year because there is a shortage of graduate-level nursing faculty.

A report by the American Association of Colleges of Nursing (AACN) shows that US nursing schools turned away 32,797 qualified applicants from baccalaureate and graduate nursing programs in 2004 due to insufficient number of faculty, clinical sites, classroom space, clinical preceptors, and budget constraints. More than 2600 applicants were turned away from nursing programs in Colorado in 2003.

Three quarters (76.1%) of the nursing schools point to faculty shortages as a reason for not accepting all qualified applicants into nursing programs. This academic year (2005–2006), 66% of nursing schools report that they have vacancies and are in need of additional nursing faculty to meet additional demand.

Colorado's shortage of qualified nursing faculty at its two-year nursing schools is three times the national average, and nearly double the national average at its four-year schools.

We anticipate this faculty shortage to escalate in the next decade due budget constraints, increased job competition from clinical sites, and the retirement of a "graying professoriate" of nursing faculty.

A wave of faculty retirements is expected within the next ten years. Between 200 and 300 doctorally-prepared faculty will be eligible for retirement each year from 2003 through 2012.

I am anxious to hear the testimony from our witnesses today. I am very proud of the collaborative efforts in Colorado to address the nursing faculty shortage. Colorado educational institutions and health care providers are working together to pursue strategies to strengthen faculty recruitment and retention.

It is my hope that we can identify some strategies to address the faculty shortage in our country. I welcome your insight so that we may work together to prepare a nursing workforce that is prepared to meet the health care needs of the nation.

––––––––

STATEMENT OF HON. JON C. PORTER, A REPRESENTATIVE IN CONGRESS FROM THE STATE OF NEVADA

Mr. PORTER. Thank you, Marilyn. I appreciate the kind and warm welcome. Certainly, coming from the great State of Nevada, I can appreciate the air and the wind is probably blowing from Nevada into Colorado. Normally we say, "What happens in Las Vegas, stays in Las Vegas," but I think maybe the winds are coming from Nevada.

But, Marilyn, I appreciate your hospitality and your friendship, but also your leadership. Marilyn and I were elected at the same time, so we were sophomores together.

Mrs. MUSGRAVE. Yes.

Mr. PORTER. We've been working closely on a number of key issues, and one that really cuts to the chase, and it has to do with the quality of life of not only residents in Colorado and Nevada, but in the country. That's health care and professionals.

To my friend, President Norton, thank you. We had a chance to meet in D.C. A few months back, talked about this very issue, and I appreciate your leadership for the State of Colorado, but also for the country. Thank you for what's happening.

I want to pick on Dan Weaver. Dan didn't make it to the airport to pick us up last night, so we had to take a cab. So, Dan, I'm sorry that you probably aren't going to have a job after today.

But in all seriousness, Dan, I appreciate your help and working with you. I know that Dan's that liaison between the process and the professionals, but also the politicians that are trying to do the right thing. So, Dan, thank you for helping out and being at the airport and getting us here safely. Thank you very much.

My staff is not with me today, so I don't have to use my notes, right? I can put these aside? I think we talked about this last night, Wanda. I just want to talk a little bit about Nevada for a moment, and then give some of my perspectives how that impacts Colorado and the rest of the country.

You know, we're experiencing very similar challenges to Colorado. We're, of course, not as large of a state, but we have the same challenges. We are one of the fastest growing states in the country. We're seeing seven, eight, nine thousand people a month moving into Nevada.

Now, I have no doubt you're experiencing similar growth, if not more, but when you look at the size of our state of about 2.2 million people, it's substantial. And we've grown almost a million people in the last decade, so that puts a lot of pressure on our infrastructure, our schools, our health care, our highways, our air quality—all of these things that we are working, and I believe quite effectively in Nevada.

But we have 18,000 new students, high school and grade school students a year. Imagine that, 18,000, and we're being two and a half new schools a month in the community of Southern Nevada. We're hiring close to 2,500 new teachers a year. We're hiring 5,000 new support staff a year into our school district.

But all of that aside, health care is right in there with the challenges. So we have multiple level of challenges. One, of course, is recruiting and finding health care professionals because of the massive growth. We need 1,000—minimum 1,000 new nurses and professionals in health care a year. A thousand. We have a shortage, really, of higher education institutions that—because we're a small state, but fortunately there's a few that have been specializing in health care.

Nevada State College, which is one of my favorite projects, it's a new college in Southern Nevada, part of the university system, that's specializing in accelerated nursing, and we've been working with President Norton and the president of the school in Henderson, Nevada, trying to learn from each other's challenges and each other's successes.

But, quality of life is really the key, and we want to make sure that Nevadans and Coloradans and the rest of the country have the absolute best health care in the world, and I believe that we have it, but there are times we have a challenge in delivering it because of a shortage.

And there's multiple ways to reach that goal, but not only do we need more educating professionals, we need, of course, more teachers that have expertise in health care. We need to make sure that our neighbors and friends and graduates, and even those looking for a change in career who want to get into the nursing profession. We want to make sure we can elevate that as a very primary role in the delivery of health care.

What's happened in the country is that we're used to now 1–800 dial-a-number, or pull it up on the web, and if you dial the 1–800 number, you have to wait or you push another number and eventually you find someone to talk to you about your health care problem. Or you go to the web or WebMD or whatever it is out there.

But American people are still begging to be taken care of and to have someone that cares. And the nursing profession and the professionals in delivery of health care, still are a good—and I'm not an expert—but 80 percent of health care is how you're treated. And I'll tell you, we need to elevate the position of nurses, find a way to make sure that they receive, one, the funding and the training and the pay that they deserve, because they play such a major— you all that are here, the professionals, play such a major role in health care. We want to make sure we continue with the best in the world, and we certainly all want to make sure if we're ill, or a friend or a relative is ill, that they receive the absolute best care.

So today is really about a lot of things, and I've learned from working with Marilyn and spending some time on this issue the last at least three full years that a key link in health care delivery is finding and encouraging professionals that would like to help teach and train.

We want to make sure that we're doing everything we can from the Federal level, and I know Marilyn and I would agree, all politics are local. We don't want to get in the way, as the Federal Government, and the Federal Government should be providing opportunities, providing incentives, but we want to make sure that the State of Colorado and the private sector and the professionals here are given the tools by the Federal Government to do what they need to do.

When I was elected, and I know when Marilyn was elected, we weren't elected to be the superintendent of schools or the president of a school, we were elected to provide support from the Federal level.

So today, I'm honored to be here, I'm excited, this is a passion for me, and I want to make sure that I can learn as much as I can from all of you and take it and share it with my community in Nevada. We're having a similar hearing in Nevada on Friday with Nevada State College, and I hope to again take some things that I've learned today and share with our folks in Nevada.

So, again, thank you very much to the school and to all of those who are here today. I'm honored, and look forward to your testimonies.

[The prepared statement of Mr. Porter follows:]

Statement of Hon. Jon C. Porter, a Representative in Congress from the State of Nevada

Good morning. Thank you all for joining us for this hearing to examine the causes and possible solutions to address the shortage of qualified nursing faculty at our nation's institutions of higher education. I'm pleased to welcome all of our witnesses here today. I appreciate you taking time out of your busy schedules to appear before the Subcommittee. I am also glad that those of you in the audience were able to attend.

As many of you know, according to the American Association of State Colleges and Universities, by 2020 experts believe there will be a national shortage of more than 800,000 registered nurses. The National League of Nursing estimates that more than 125,000 qualified applicants were rejected by nursing programs in the 2003–2004 academic year. The shortage of nursing faculty is one of several factors that are most commonly cited as reasons behind this trend.

This problem is even more severe in the state of Nevada, where I am from, than in some other states. In fact, according to the U.S. Department of Health and Human Services' National Center for Health Workforce Analysis, Nevada's projected shortage of nurses will increase from 11% in 2000 to 27.5% in 2020.

While I am troubled by the magnitude of this problem, and its impact on our nation I am also hopeful that the testimony we hear today will provide us with some additional insights as to what can be done to address the issue. I look forward to hearing more from our witnesses about the challenges our nation is facing and what is being done to find solutions.

I believe that this national crisis must be confronted with coordinated efforts at the federal, state, and local levels. While the federal government must work harder to provide the resources to enhance the ability to train nurses, state and local governments, as well as private entities, will play a major role in reversing the declines in the nursing workforce. The national health implications of this dilemma are too serious, and the cost to patients too great to remain inactive. We must continue to look to build relationships and develop plans of action that will address these problems in a comprehensive manner. Through hearings like this, and the continued efforts of schools of nursing, we can educate Members of Congress as to how we can best overcome these issues.

I'd also like to take this opportunity to thank Congresswoman Marilyn Musgrave for her interest in this issue, and her invitation to come to Greeley to discuss this issue further.—I look forward to working with her as we continue to examine what can be done at all levels of government to address the shortage of qualified nursing faculty.

Again, thank you for joining us today to provide your valuable insight into this most important issue. I look forward to continuing our work to alleviate the pressures currently being placed on the nursing workforce.

———

Mrs. MUSGRAVE. Thank you, Jon, very much.

Our first witness today is Ms. Sue Carparelli. She's the president and chief executive officer of the Colorado Center for Nursing Excellence in Denver. Ms. Carparelli has a background in both workforce development and health care, and is spearheading the only collaborative statewide initiative to improve access to quality health care through the development and support of Colorado's nursing workforce.

She also works on a wide variety of educational issues, with a special emphasis on the nursing shortage. Thank you for being here, and we're looking forward to hearing from you.

You know, when we're in Washington, D.C., we have a very prominent light that limits you to 5 minutes, but we're going to be merciful. We don't have the light, so we're just going to guess at it. Thank you very much.

STATEMENT OF SUE CARPARELLI, PRESIDENT AND CEO, COLORADO CENTER FOR NURSING EXCELLENCE, DENVER, CO

Ms. CARPARELLI. Thank you. Thank you. I will attempt to keep that light in my eyes nevertheless, and I want to thank you very much for being here. We are very grateful for your attention to what we think is a very important issue as well. As I look around this room, I'm also humble in my having the opportunity to speak to you, because there are many, many experts in this room who could provide a great deal of information on this issue for you. But let me see if I can't summarize some of the key issues from our perspective.

First, the Center for Nursing Excellence is an independent, nonprofit organization. It was established in 2002 to be working as a convener, broker, facilitator of solution building in our state as we address nursing workforce issues. As such, we have the opportunity to work with many stakeholder groups across the state and have learned a great deal about what works and doesn't work in that process.

The Center's funding comes from industry investment, it comes from state and Federal grants and foundation grants.

First of all, let me just put some things in context for you as we then focus more specifically on the nursing faculty shortage.

Health care in our state is a very important economic engine, and I think it would be critical that we keep that in focus as we consider the communities large and small, rural and urban, across our state.

One in 10 Coloradans work in health care, and the health care sector is expected to create more jobs than any other industry sector in Colorado over the next decade, yet the efficiency of the engine is stymied by shortages. The Department of Labor in our state predicts that more than 7,300 health care jobs will go unfilled each year for the next decade because there will not be enough workers prepared to meet that demand.

Registered nurses in our state make up 25 percent of that health care work force, and you talked about the shortages in our state and the rate of growth that is projected by 2020 to be about a 31 percent shortage.

This shortage in our state, as in other states, results from the interplay of both supply side and demand side factors. First, we are losing nurses faster than we can produce them. They are old. The average age of nurses——

Mr. PORTER. You'd better be careful.

Ms. CARPARELLI.—in Colorado—I know, I know, but I'm—we're going to talk honestly here. Average age in our state of Colorado nurses is 47 years old.

Importantly, it is essential that you note that only 7 percent of our nursing workforce is under 30. So the point in that is that we are missing essentially an entire generation of nurses.

We also have a mismatch of diversity. The racial and ethnic make-up of our current nursing workforce does not reflect the increasing diversity of the state. Only 7.6 percent of Colorado nurses are nonwhite. Of that, 3 percent are Hispanic, while we are a state that has about 16 percent of our population of Hispanic descent.

You have referenced the fact that nurses are predominantly women. In our state, that is 95 percent. We have not seen men enter this profession at the same rate as we have seen women leave it.

Against this backdrop, we face an aging population whose health care needs will only increase in the years to come, placing more stress on an already overburdened system.

As you referenced, our state is one that is growing. By 2020, Colorado's total population is expected to grow by 16 percent with 113 percent growth in our population of persons age 65 and over. That becomes a critical factor in considering demand for health care.

Our efforts to increase the supply of registered nurses to meet this demand are greatly complicated by an education system that struggles to produce enough graduates to replace our diminishing and aging work force.

While we enjoy a large supply of willing students, and you've noted both nationally and our state, that we are not able to respond to the number of people who are interested in entering this profession because of a variety of factors.

The No. 1 reason for this trend in our ability to absorb those who are interested in entering this profession has to do with the insufficient numbers of qualified faculty to meet the demand of prospective students.

In our state, as in other areas, the faculty shortage is most acute among clinical faculty, and those are the nursing educators who oversee students' hands on learning experiences at the bedside, which is a very essential component of nursing education.

My colleague, Lynn Dierker, will tell you more about the reasons and implications and some of the specific solutions in terms of Colorado's nursing faculty shortage based on a study that was recently completed by the Colorado Health Institute. But let me make some additional observations in relation to the findings that you'll hear from her.

First, in our state, we have at this point, I think, an unprecedented level of collaboration amongst our schools of nursing and amongst the faculty and leaders within those schools. This is affording us an opportunity to learn from one another, to look at best practices, and to share those ideas which work best.

An information clearing house, on a national basis for best practices on nursing education and faculty development, is also crucial. And models such as that outlined by the University of Northern Colorado's proposal for the National Center for Nursing Education, offering coordination and technical assistance, resources, and professional development for nursing educators, is an excellent way to continue this work on a national level.

Second, we can address the shortage of clinical leaning opportunities, in part, by taking advantage of emerging technologies, new opportunities and methods for learning. Colorado is poised to become a national leader in the effective use of those technologies, and we are grateful for the leadership that has been provided by the Colorado Department of Labor, which led to funding of a new collaborative simulation center, which will be on the Fitzsimons Campus; that project being funded by the U.S. Department of Labor.

The Colorado Center for Nursing Excellence has been charged to operate this new resource, which will make the state-of-the-art patient simulation resources available to students and faculty from around the state—in particular, to help develop the capacity of faculty to use these new technologies.

And third, we have found that clinical practitioners, those clinical experts practicing within the health care delivery system, are willing partner in education when we provide them preparation and support to perform the clinical instructor role.

We have been benefited in our state by a grant through the Colorado Department of Labor, which has allowed us to develop and proliferate what's referred to as a clinical scholar model. This trains practicing nurses to become clinical scholars, overseeing the rotations at practice sites, and the response to this particular program has been extremely gratifying. We have filled out grant-funded slots and nurses continue to be interested in these roles and we are seeing industry—in other words, the employers, particular in the acute care setting, support the cost of their participation.

We are looking next at creating a statewide inventory of both supply and demand of clinical sites. This is another element that's contributing to our inability to support student learning. And what we believe is that we have the opportunity to create a technology platform that will support, then, that information enabling us to have a better sense and more efficient use of what is also a scarce resource in terms of clinical sites.

These examples and others, which will be noted by Elise Lowe-Vaughn from the Department of Labor, illustrate the role of state and Federal agencies in addressing Colorado's and the nation's nursing faculty shortage.

While the Colorado Center for Nursing Excellence is fortunate to have strong support from Colorado's hospital and foundation community, ongoing Federal support and investment in efforts such as ours across the country, is essential.

Agencies, such as the U.S. Department of Labor and the Department of Health and Human Services, play an integral role in solving our nursing labor shortage.

In closing, I wish to draw the community's attention to one inescapable fact: Health care workers are knowledge workers. While many of those currently employed within the health care sector are prepared through on-the-job training programs, generally funded by employers, nursing requires highly specialized and costly education and lifelong learning opportunities which are accessible only through our colleges and universities.

In order to prepare these essential health care workers, we must have a viable, accessible, educational system that is responsive to the evolving needs of current health care practice.

And I welcome any questions that you have, and thank you for this opportunity.

Mrs. MUSGRAVE. That was very excellent testimony.

[The prepared statement of Ms. Carparelli follows:]

Statement of Sue Carparelli, President & CEO, Colorado Center for Nursing Excellence, Denver, CO

Thank you, members of the Committee. My name is Sue Carparelli; I am president and chief executive officer of the Colorado Center for Nursing Excellence.

The Center is an independent, nonprofit organization established in 2002. It is the only organization in Colorado exclusively dedicated to ensuring that our state has adequate numbers of highly-qualified nurses. We bring together educational institutions, health care providers, governmental agencies and foundations to investigate the sources of the nursing shortfall, to develop strategies to address it and to secure resources needed for effective solution building. The Center serves as a source of information and technical assistance, a broker and convener of collaborative partnerships and as a catalyst for innovation.

Center funding comes from industry investments, grants from federal and state agencies, and foundation grants.

My purpose today is to support my colleagues in illuminating the factors contributing to Colorado's shortage of qualified nursing faculty, and help them and members of this committee explore solutions to this crucial problem.

I would like to begin my remarks by creating context around Colorado's nursing faculty shortage. I will provide some important facts about Colorado's healthcare workforce, and explain our state's nursing shortage. Then I will explore the impact of the shortage of nursing faculty on our ability to fill the nursing gap. I will furnish examples of efforts the Colorado Center for Nursing Excellence has underway to alleviate the faculty shortage, and offer recommendations to the Committee as you consider the federal government's role in addressing this nationwide problem.

Healthcare is an economic engine in Colorado. One in 10 Coloradans work in healthcare, and the healthcare sector is expected to create more jobs than any other industry sector in Colorado over the next decade.

Yet, the efficiency of that engine is stymied by shortages. The Colorado Department of Labor predicts that more than 7300 healthcare jobs will go unfilled each year for the next decade because there will not be enough workers prepared to meet the demand.

The shortage is especially acute among registered nurses. Members of the committee are already, I am sure, well aware of the nationwide nursing shortage. Colorado's shortage is especially dire.

While registered nurses currently make up 25 percent of all healthcare workers in our state, Colorado is estimated to have about 5,000 fewer nurses than we need, or a 13 percent shortfall. That's about double the national average. And, that figure is expected to grow to 31 percent—or nearly 17,000 fewer nurses than needed in Colorado—by 2020 if current trends continue. This shortfall results from the interplay of both supply side and demand side factors.

First, we are losing nurses faster than we produce them. The average age of a Colorado hospital nurse is currently 47. Only 7 percent are under age 30. A 2003 study found that 45 percent of Colorado nurses did not expect to be practicing in five years.

Further, the racial and ethnic makeup of the current nursing workforce does not reflect the increasing diversity of the state. Only 7.6 percent of Colorado nurses are non-white; 3 percent are Hispanic, in a state whose population is nearly 16 percent Hispanic.

In addition, women have left nursing for other professions and few men have entered the profession to take their place. Today, 95 percent of Colorado nurses are female, while only 5 percent are male.

Against this backdrop, we face—as do all other states—an aging population whose healthcare needs will only increase in the years to come, placing still more stress on an already overburdened system. Our population is also growing. By 2020, Colorado's total population is expected to grow 16 percent, with 113 percent growth among those age 65 and older.

Our efforts to increase the supply of registered nurses to meet this demand are greatly complicated by a higher education system that is failing to produce enough graduates to replace our diminishing, aging workforce. While we enjoy a large supply of willing students, our nursing education programs are severely constrained by a lack of qualified faculty.

From a national perspective, it is important—and somewhat disheartening—to note that Colorado's nursing faculty shortage is typical, not unique. A study earlier this year by the American Association of Colleges of Nursing found that nursing schools around the country rejected 32,000 qualified students in 2004, despite a 14 percent gain in enrollment from the previous year. In Colorado in 2003 (the most recent year for which data are available), 2600 qualified applicants were turned away from nursing programs. The number one reason for this disturbing trend is that Colorado's nursing schools, as well as those elsewhere in the country, simply do not have sufficient numbers of faculty to meet the demand from prospective students.

Our faculty shortage is most acute among clinical faculty, the professionals who oversee student nurses' hands-on experiences at the bedside. The bottleneck for clinical rotations means that nursing students wait longer for placements and have less time on rotations once they secure them. This essential element in nurse preparation, and one which is especially critical for developing the observation and treatment skills necessary to providing high quality care, is thus jeopardized.

My colleague Lynn Dierker will tell you more about the reasons for, implications of, and specific solutions to Colorado's nursing faculty shortage, based on a recent study conducted by the Colorado Health Institute under the Center's auspices. I want to set the stage for her comments by making a few observations of my own.

First, our nursing schools must have opportunities to learn from each others' successes and tap into the latest thinking on nurse education. An information clearinghouse for best practices on nursing education and faculty development is crucial. The model outlined in the University of Northern Colorado's proposal for the National Center for Nursing Education, offering coordination, technical assistance, resources and professional development for nursing educators, is an excellent way to fill this need.

Second, we can address the shortage of clinical learning opportunities, in part, by taking advantage of emerging simulation technologies. In fact, Colorado is posed to become a national leader in the effective use of these technologies. The U.S. Department of Labor recently awarded funds to the Colorado Dept. of Labor and Employment to create the Work, Education and Lifelong Learning Simulation Center, known as the WELLS Center. The Colorado Center for Nursing Excellence is overseeing this important new resource, which will make state-of-the art patient simulation resources accessible to students and faculty from around the state through high-speed datacasting.

Third, and perhaps most encouraging, we have found that clinical practitioners become more willing to oversee student rotations when the practitioners are trained in how to fill that role. Indeed, practicing nurses have signed up eagerly for a new training program provided by the Colorado Center for Nursing Excellence under a grant from the Colorado Department of Labor and Employment. This Faculty Development Project trains practicing nurses to become "clinical scholars," overseeing student rotations at practice sites throughout Colorado. Response to the program has been so overwhelming that the grant-funded slots were filled long ago, yet nurses continue to sign up for the opportunity, with their institutions covering the cost of their participation.

The Colorado Center for Nursing Excellence is also poised to develop a statewide inventory of both the supply and demand for clinical teaching sites, supported by a technology platform which will enable efficient matching based on tailored selection criteria. We are currently seeking funding for this initiative.

These examples—and others that will be noted by my colleague Tom Looft from the Colorado Department of Labor—all illustrate the role of state and federal agencies in addressing Colorado's, and the nation's, nursing faculty shortage. While the Colorado Center for Nursing Excellence is fortunate to have strong support from Colorado's hospital and foundation community, ongoing federal support and investment is essential for our efforts—and similar programs around the country—to be successful. Agencies such as the U.S. Department of Labor and the Department of Health and Human Services play an integral role in solving our nursing labor shortage, providing the funds that fuel good ideas.

In closing, I wish to draw the committee's attention to one inescapable fact. Healthcare workers are knowledge workers. While many of those currently employed within the healthcare sector are prepared through on the job training programs generally funded by employers, nursing requires highly specialized and costly education and training accessible only through our colleges and universities. In order to prepare these essential health care workers we must have a viable, accessible educational system that is responsive to the evolving needs of current health care practice.

I welcome any questions from the committee. Thank you.

Mrs. MUSGRAVE. I think we'll hear from all of the witnesses and then we'll come back for questions.

Ms. CARPARELLI. Thank you.

Mrs. MUSGRAVE. That was very good.

Our next witness is Ms. Lynn Dierker. She's an R.N. Who currently serves as the deputy director for community initiatives at the Colorado Health Institute, and she holds a bachelor of science in nursing from Emory University, and a bachelor of arts from Drew University.

As deputy director for community initiatives, she is responsible for building sustained partnerships for distancing nursing education between the institute and its diverse constituents throughout the state. Welcome.

STATEMENT OF LYNN DIERKER, R.N., DIRECTOR FOR COMMUNITY INITIATIVES, COLORADO HEALTH INSTITUTE, DENVER, CO

Ms. DIERKER. Thank you very much. I appreciate the opportunity to speak to you today.

The Colorado Health Institute is an independent 501(C)(3) created by three foundations in Colorado to be an independent source of information, objective nonpartial information, for policymakers at both community and statewide levels.

I'm here today to provide brief highlights from the 2004 study that we completed related to the Colorado nursing workforce and the shortage of nursing faculty. And we completed this at the request of the Colorado Center for Nursing Excellent, and with funding by the Colorado State Workforce Council.

A copy of the entire study is provided to you, and I think you have one with you there today——

Mrs. MUSGRAVE. Yes.

Ms. DIERKER.—and I recommend it as a rich resource of information. However, during the next few minutes, I hope to put into context the key findings from the study and discuss their implications, particularly as you consider how best to partner with states to promote nursing workforce development. As I make my few remarks here today, I don't know about you, but in listening to study findings, it's awfully difficult to hear data rattled off. So, what I've done is really refer you to the study for specific numbers and findings, and I'm going to try and this sort of the key concepts and implications of the findings in the study.

The study was designed to identify and analyze key factors and issues affecting the supply of and demand for nursing faculty; in particular, the relationship between nurse education programs and the market for nurses and the health care industry.

The study focuses on four primary areas: Economic factors, non-economic factors, education infrastructure, and the role played by the private sector. And the study included issues related to both licensed practical nursing and registered nursing education programs.

The research we did took full advantage of what is available in the current nursing workforce literature, and we also collected primary data through two Web-based surveys; one of clinical sites that employ nurses and train them, and one of educational programs across our state. We also interviewed many key informants from both practice and education and used an advisory panel to advise us on our study design and methodology.

So, as to our key findings, let me put these in the context of what you're already hearing about the national workforce shortage and faculty shortages, and what you've already heard today about Colorado's situation.

Our current nurse faculty shortage is significantly greater than the national average, as you've heard. The national shortage of faculty being around 8.6 percent, our shortages range from 15 percent in our 4 year institutions to 25 percent among our 2 year programs, including, importantly, our community colleges.

In the face of this nationwide shortage, Colorado struggles to compete with other states to attract faculty due to these economic and noneconomic factors, including compensation levels, workload demands, and budget constraints that disproportionately affect our state-supported higher education.

With population growth, as you've heard, and increasing demand for nursing services, Colorado, like other states, has called upon its education system to produce greater numbers of nursing graduates. The study found that nursing education deployed significant and rapid program expansions over the past 3 years. However, in a number of ways, these expansions exacerbated our faculty shortage and increased job dissatisfaction.

Entry-level faculty salaries are low; less than $40,000 on average, and even less in rural areas, and especially related to available positions within clinical institutions offering greatly higher rates of pay.

Workloads are heavy, especially for clinical instructors who most often work on an hourly contract basis without benefits.

In this context, concerns, as you've mentioned, are growing about faculty attrition due to retirements which are projected to increase significantly due to the average age of Colorado faculty, 50, especially within the state's 4 year colleges and universities.

Preparing adequate numbers of qualified faculty is another corollary issue. The study reveals a lack of incentives and opportunities for graduate level preparation for nurses interested in a teaching role. Anecdotally, we heard from many who report that nurses who are in clinical settings and interested in taking on faculty roles can't afford the time and the resources to go full time to an education program and to have access to graduate level preparation.

The majority of the state's nursing programs in Colorado are publicly funded and are, therefore, caught up in the current fiscal crisis facing all of higher education in our state. The study found that the private sector, particularly those clinical facilities employing newly graduated nurses, in particular, hospitals and long-term care facilities, private sectors already spending millions of dollars per year to support nursing education.

However, clinical facilities report that newly graduated nurses are often unprepared to assume the full responsibilities of independent practice and they, therefore, require continuing training and supports that range again to the tune of millions of dollars annually.

In addition to providing examples of widespread stress and concern related to faculty shortages, our study informants provided a rich picture of the types of innovation that are beginning to take hold within nursing education. As Sue has mentioned, these include advances in technology to enhance teaching methods and collaborative relationships with clinical facilities to strengthen the level of preparedness of new graduates and improve faculty job satisfaction. The study found that Colorado's nursing programs and health care facilities are pursuing many of the promising strategies that we identified nationally and by other states.

CHI was charged to provide timely information that would support stakeholder decisionmaking about opportunities and investments in programs and interventions. This study is a starting point. It's a snapshot in time, and highlights the need for more robust, well-defined, and reliable data monitoring efforts by which to understand the full picture of nursing workforce supply and demand over time.

However, the findings make it clear that Colorado educators, clinical training sites, and policymakers face both substantial challenges and exciting opportunities related to strengthening not only the nursing workforce, but also the healthcare system as a whole.

In conclusion, I want to offer observations regarding the important three-level partnership that exists between Federal, state, and local leaders and policymakers. At the community level, even in our rural areas, nursing educators and clinicians perceive the need for strategic alignment of goals and strategies to meet the healthcare challenges before us. Study informants note that many of the issues related to nursing workforce, and particularly faculty development, should be addressed by a policy framework and resources made available at the national level.

At the same time, as a system in need of innovation, nursing education must rely on and have the support for creativity and the ability to be responsive at the local and state system level among institutions, and with leadership that nurse practice and education leaders provide.

Collaboration, flexibility, funding, and strategic and sustained alignment of efforts are themes that emerge from this study, and are offered for your consideration.

Again, I am grateful for the opportunity to present this very brief overview, and welcome any questions or comments you may have. Thank you.

Mrs. MUSGRAVE. Thank you. We'll have questions for you a little later, I'm sure.

[The prepared statement of Ms. Dierker follows:]

Statement of Lynn Dierker, R.N., Director for Community Institute, Colorado Health Institute, Denver, CO

Thank you for the opportunity to speak to you today. My name is Lynn Dierker. I am Director for Community Initiatives with the Colorado Health Institute.

The Colorado Health Institute is an independent 501(c)(3) created by three Colorado foundations to be an information resource for policy makers at both community and state levels. CHI's mission is to improve the health of Coloradans through informed decision making. To carry out this mission, CHI works to improve the availability of data, conduct policy research and analysis, and perhaps most importantly, facilitate the dissemination of information so that it is used most effectively to understand and address the pressing issues affecting our communities and our state. As an organization, CHI is distinct in its independence and ability to serve as a neutral convener, bringing together stakeholders with diverse perspectives to work collaboratively to collect, analyze, and discuss data and their implications for health improvement in our state.

I am here to provide brief highlights from a 2004 study of Colorado's nursing workforce and the shortage of nursing faculty that CHI completed at the request of the Colorado Center for Nursing Excellence. A copy of the entire study is being provided to you as a resource. However, during the next few minutes I hope to put into context key findings from the study and discuss their implications, particularly as you consider how best to partner with states to promote nursing workforce development.

The Colorado Nursing Faculty Supply and Demand Study (Study) was designed to identify and analyze key factors and issues affecting the supply of and demand for nursing faculty, including the relationship between nurse education programs and the market for professional nurses in Colorado. The Study focuses on four primary areas: 1) economic factors including the economic rewards of teaching; 2) non-economic factors such as faculty workload, work environment, opportunities for professional development, and faculty educational requirements; 3) the infrastructure of Colorado nurse education programs; and 4) the role played by the private sector. The Study examined issues related to both licensed practical nursing (LPN) and registered nursing (RN) educational programs.

The research effort took full advantage of information available in the current nursing workforce literature, and also collected primary data from Colorado nursing programs and clinical training sites related to the recruitment and retention of nursing faculty. An advisory panel of experts informed the study design and methodology.

I want to highlight key findings from the Study in the context of what you are learning about nursing workforce issues nationwide. Colorado's current nurse faculty shortage is significantly greater than the national average shortage of 8.6 %, with shortages ranging from 15% in our four year institutions, to 25% among two year institutions including community colleges.

In the face of a nationwide shortage, Colorado struggles to compete with other states to attract faculty due to economic and non-economic factors including compensation levels, workload demands and budget constraints that disproportionately affect state-supported higher education.

With population growth and increasing demand for nursing services, Colorado, like other states, has called upon its education system to produce greater numbers of nursing graduates. The Study found that nursing education deployed significant and rapid program expansions over the past three years in response to the workforce shortage. However, in a number of ways, these expansions exacerbated the faculty shortage and increased job dissatisfaction. Entry level faculty salaries are low, especially related to available positions within clinical institutions at higher rates of pay. Work loads are heavy especially for clinical instructors who most often work on a hourly contract basis without benefits. In this context, concerns are growing about faculty attrition due to retirements, which are projected to increase significantly due to the average age of Colorado faculty, especially within the state's four year colleges and universities. Preparing adequate numbers of qualified faculty is another corollary issue. The Study reveals a lack of incentives and opportunities for graduate level preparation for nurses interested in a teaching role.

The majority of the state's nursing programs are publicly funded and are therefore caught up in the current fiscal crisis facing all of higher education in Colorado. The Study found that the private sector, particularly clinical facilities employing newly graduated nurses (hospitals and long term care facilities), is already spending millions of dollars per year to support nursing education. This support takes the form of subsidizing clinical faculty; providing clinical instruction; offering scholarships and tuition reimbursement; and expanding clinical rotations to meet the increased demand for clinical training sites. However, clinical facilities report that newly graduated nurses are often unprepared to assume the responsibilities of independent practice. Concerns over the quality of patient care require them to provide orientation programs to new graduates ranging from four weeks to greater than three months and costing in excess of $2 million dollars annually.

In addition to providing examples of widespread stress and concern related to faculty shortages, Study informants provided a rich picture of the types of innovation beginning to take hold within nursing education. These include advances in technology to enhance teaching methods, and collaborative relationships with clinical facilities to strengthen the level of preparedness of new graduates and improve faculty job satisfaction. Nursing programs have begun to utilize technology to enhance existing teaching methods and the overall educational experience. Together with clinical training sites, educational programs are striving to develop sustainable collaborative approaches to strengthen the competencies of new nurse graduates. The challenges inherent in these innovative projects are how to successfully achieve technology transfer and ensure widespread adoption of those practices that yield the best results.

The findings from this study point to the need for coordinated and strategic action. A solid foundation of public and private sector collaboration has been established. Reporting new levels of partnership, Colorado's nursing programs and health care facilities are pursuing many of the most promising strategies identified nationally and by other states, particularly related to cultivating an adequate supply of clinical faculty. Colorado-specific initiatives designed to support and strengthen faculty roles and resources are emerging.

There are additional opportunities to further the use of non-traditional and multi-disciplinary approaches to faculty development such as streamlining graduate program requirements, use of interdisciplinary faculty teams, and expansion of regional institutional collaborations. Regulatory and institutional policies warrant further examination related to the continuum of educational opportunities for practicing nurses including opportunities to better utilize Colorado's pool of retired nurse educators.

As Study informants note, nurse faculty issues are inexorably linked to the complex range of factors that contribute to the overall nursing workforce shortage. Other states offer approaches for recruiting and training nurse educators that Colorado should consider. State experiences suggest that it is necessary to dig below the surface to address fundamental components of a transformed 21st health care system that can deliver quality health care in a cost-effective manner. These key questions must be answered by each state, but also collectively. What are the numbers and qualifications of nurse educators that are needed? What array of nursing education programs is needed to yield the right mix of practicing nurses? What data is needed to inform these decisions?

CHI was charged to provide timely information that would support stakeholder decision-making about opportunities and investments in programs and interventions. This study is a starting point for understanding both the contributing factors and potential solutions for Colorado's nurse faculty shortages. It is a snapshot in time and highlights the need for more robust, well-defined and reliable data monitoring efforts by which to understand the full picture of nursing workforce supply and demand over time and the factors associated with affecting noted trends. However, the findings make it clear that Colorado educators, clinical training sites and policy makers face both substantial challenges and exciting opportunities related to strengthening not only the nursing workforce, but also the health care system as a whole.

In conclusion, I want to offer observations regarding the important three-way partnership that exists between federal, state and local leaders and policy makers. At the community level, even in rural areas, nursing educators and clinicians perceive the need for strategic alignment of goals and strategies to meet the health care challenges before us. Study informants note that many of the issues related to nursing workforce and particularly faculty development should be addressed by a policy framework and resources made available at the national level. At the same time, as a system in need of innovation, nursing education must rely on the creativity and responsiveness of local and state systems, institutions, and leaders. Collaboration, flexibility, funding, and strategic and sustained alignment of efforts are themes that emerged from this Study and are offered for your consideration.

I welcome any questions or comments from the committee. Thank you!

———

Mrs. MUSGRAVE. Our next witness is Elise Lowe-Vaughn, and she's the operations director for the workforce programs and the Colorado Department of Labor and Employment. She has an undergraduate degree in humanities and has done graduate work in counseling. She also helped to develop a multilevel computer literacy curricula for the Electronic Colorado Learning Portal that targets the hardest to serve and adult education participants. Thank you for being here.

STATEMENT OF ELISE LOWE-VAUGHN, OPERATIONS DIRECTOR, WORKFORCE DEVELOPMENT PROGRAMS, COLORADO DEPARTMENT OF LABOR AND EMPLOYMENT, DENVER, CO

Ms. LOWE-VAUGHN. Thank you, Members of the Committee. I'm honored to speak with you today about the nursing shortage and its impact on our economy and the variety of nursing and faculty initiatives funded by the Colorado Department of Labor and Employment and the Colorado State Workforce Development Council.

Colorado's workforce system is a national leader because of its unique collaborative partnerships, its innovation, and its ability to embrace the emerging technologies to meet industries demands in critical workforce occupations.

Worker shortages in healthcare occupations, particularly in nursing, have been the focus of Federal, state, and local initiatives the past several years.

In Colorado, during the past 3 years, the Colorado Department of Labor and Employment and the State Workforce Development Council, have funded over $3 million in discretionary workforce investment act and Wagner-Peyser projects that are targeted at improving the supply of nurses and allied healthcare professionals and providing career ladders to support advancement opportunity, and also faculty development opportunities.

Some examples of the projects that have been funded include scholarships to upgrade bachelors and graduate-level nurses, recruitment of minority and youth populations into the profession, development of assessment tools to support students' ability to succeed in nursing programs, remediation programs to mentor high-risk nursing students, expansion of clinical rotationsites, the creation of associates and bachelors degrees in rural areas, and the state community colleges' nursing program accreditation.

Concurrently, the Department, acting as a neutral convener of industry leaders and educational institutions, held forums around the state to identify creative approaches to the nursing shortage so that we could positively effect the nursing supply pipeline.

We solicited the Center for Nursing Excellence to develop the Colorado nursing faculty supply and demand study. The findings from the study, and the results of the various forums around the state, highlighted the need to take the statewide system building approach to nursing and faculty development.

From these conversations, the idea for the Work, Education, and Life-long Learning Simulation Center was spawned and a grant was requested and funded from the U.S. Department of Labor. This technology-based public-private venture weaves together the insights learned from the past 3 years, and has helped us identify a 5-year multiphase course of action.

The center will be located at the Fitzsimons Redevelopment Center, and the space was contributed in part from the University of Colorado Hospital and partially funded from the state. This center will probably be the most sophisticated clinical training facility in the country for nurses and for nursing faculty.

In the first year, we have purchased over a million dollars of state-of-the-art equipment. The center will harness various technologies and employ a variety of procedure-specific simulations that meld virtual reality and computerized simulation, and transmit these via the airwaves using the public broadcast system's data casting. It is anticipated that this national demonstration will expand the depth and breadth of statewide healthcare training, and be a template for replication around the country.

Partners in this grant included Department of Labor and Employment, the State Workforce Council, the University of Colorado Hospital, the Center for Nursing Excellence, Touch of Life, the Rocky Mountain Public Broadcast System, the University of Colorado Health Sciences Simulation Center, the Colorado Area Health Education Center, and all of the collaborations of the many healthcare industry leaders, as well as educational facilities around the state. And we have over 55 partners involved in this, and it is a statewide grant.

Deeply embedded in the state's holistic strategy for expanding and improving the number, the quality, and the quantity of nursing professionals is the nursing faculty development grant. We funded this grant with the Center for Nursing Excellence with a four-to-one match from our industry and educational partners. This initiative seeks to increase the number of clinical scholars, clinical instructors, classroom instructors, lecturers, and preceptors.

Through this 2 year, million dollars project, subject matter experts have partnered to develop curricula and train clinical scholars and preceptors in the use of simulation technology to enhance skill-based competencies.

The Department's workforce learning management system will be a repository for statewide and natural virtual mentor clearing house for faculty development support.

The aforementioned approaches to this health care crisis are examples of what the state workforce development system has developed in response to President Bush's call for innovative workforce solutions, built and sustained through strategic partnerships.

Critical to all of our efforts are the public-private collaborative partnerships, which all of us have been talking about. Though they present unprecedented challenges for government and its processes, these unique initiatives afford us the opportunity to confront the status quo and build for the future.

Mrs. MUSGRAVE. Thank you very much for your testimony.

[The prepared statement of Ms. Lowe-Vaughn follows:]

Statement of Elise Lowe–Vaughn, Operations Director, Workforce Development Programs, Colorado Department of Labor and Employment, Denver, CO

Thank you members of the Committee, I am honored to speak with you today. My name is Elise Lowe–Vaughn; I am the Operations Director for Workforce Programs at the Colorado Department of Labor and Employment

Being competitive in today's global economy requires innovative workforce solutions. In 2003, the Miliken Institute ranked Colorado third in the nation for future technology growth. I am here today to speak to the variety of nursing and faculty initiatives funded by the Colorado Department of Labor and Employment (CDLE) and the Colorado State Workforce Development Council (CSWDC). These initiatives have been targeted to meet industry demands for critical workforce occupations and employ emerging technology-based solutions. Worker shortages in healthcare occupations, particularly in nursing, have been the focus of federal, state and local workforce initiatives the past few years.

In Colorado, during the last three years, the CDLE and the CSWDC funded over three million dollars in Discretionary Workforce Investment Act (WIA) and Wagner–Peyser (WP) projects targeted at improving the supply of nurses and allied healthcare professionals, providing career ladders to support advancement opportunities, and faculty development opportunities. Funds were competitively awarded to regional workforce development programs that partnered with industry and education to develop locally driven solutions to their healthcare worker shortages. Grantees were required to have partners that brought non-federal in-kind or matching funds. Grant funds were intended to seed initiatives that would directly affect change at the local, community level. Examples of projects funded include: Scholarships to upgrade two year, four year and graduate level Nurses; recruitment of minority populations and youth into healthcare professions; development of assessment tools geared to assess an individual's readiness to handle the rigors of nursing education programs; remediation programs to mentor high-risk nursing students; expansion of clinical rotation sites; creation of Associate and Bachelor degreed programs for nurses in rural areas of the state; and accreditation of the State's Community College Nursing Programs.

Concurrently, the CDLE and the CSWDC, acting as neutral conveners of industry leaders and educational institutions, held healthcare forums around the State to identify creative approaches to the nursing shortage that could positively impact the nursing supply pipeline. The CSWDC also solicited the Center for Nursing Excellence (CNE) to develop the Colorado Nursing Faculty Supply and Demand Study. The findings from this study, and the results from the various forums and funded initiatives, highlighted the need to take a statewide system-building approach to nursing and faculty development rather than using individual initiatives that weren't able to be replicated on a grand scale or didn't have the momentum to ameliorate the healthcare worker shortages.

Galvanized by the results of the statewide healthcare forums, the Nursing Faculty Supply and Demand Study, and the locally funded CDLE and CSWDC initiatives, many within the healthcare community, have come to see the value added by public/private alliances.

These conversations spawned the idea for a grant request to the US Department of Labor (USDOL) to create the Work, Education and Lifelong Learning Simulation (WELLS) Center. This technology-based public/private joint venture weaves together the insights learned over the past three years, and has helped us identify a five-year, multi-phased course of action. The WELLS Center will be located at the Fitzsimons Redevelopment Center in space contributed by the University of Colorado Hospital, and partially funded by CDLE and CSWDC. It took over eighteen months to conceive the design framework for the Center; and it will be one of the most sophisticated clinical training facilities in the country for nurses and nursing faculty.

USDOL funded this national model in phases, with first-year funds targeted at purchasing a million dollars of state-of-the-art equipment. The Center will harness various technologies and employ a variety of procedure specific simulators that meld virtual reality and computerized simulation, and transmit this learning via the air waves using high-speed data-casting. Through the use of technology, students can build their clinical competencies without risk or harm to patients, and faculty can hone their teaching skills using cutting edge systems.

The WELLS Center grant was submitted to USDOL by the CDLE and CSWDC, and represents a partnership on a grand scale among government, education, the public broadcast system, and industry competitors. Industry and non-federal partners contributed a two-to-one in-kind fund match for all federal funds invested into the grant. It is anticipated that this national demonstration will expand the depth and breadth of statewide healthcare training and be a template for replication around the country. This alignment of resources will afford all a benefit beyond their individual means. Partners in the grant included:

Colorado Department of Labor and Employment
Colorado State Workforce Development Council
University of Colorado Hospital
Center for Nursing Excellence
Touch of Life
Rocky Mountain Public Broadcasting System
University of Colorado Health Sciences Simulation Center
Colorado Area Health Education Centers

In addition, investors and collaborators in the Nursing Faculty Development Initiative and Simulation Development Group that played key roles in this process included:

Adams State College
Banner Health
Centura Health Systems
Colorado Community College System
Colorado Permanente Medical Group
Columbine Health System
Craig Hospital
Denver Health Medical Center
Emily Griffith Opportunity School
Exempla Healthcare
HealthONE
Kaiser Permanente
Mesa State College
Metropolitan State College of Denver
Platt College
Poudre Valley Hospital
Regis University–Loretto Heights Department of Nursing
University of Colorado at Denver and Health Sciences Center

University of Colorado, Colorado Springs
Beth El College of Nursing and Health Sciences
University of Northern Colorado
T.H. Pickens Technical Center
San Luis Valley Regional Medical Center
St. Mary's Hospital

We have learned that the nursing shortage is compounded by a deficit of clinical practitioners and faculty needed to train the additional number of nurse needed to meet the nation's healthcare needs. Deeply embedded in the State's holistic strategy for expanding and improving the number, the quality and the quantity of nursing professionals is the Nursing Faculty Development Grant. Funded by the CDLE, with a four-to-one in-kind match from our industry and educational partners, this initiative seeks to increase the number of clinical scholars, clinical instructors, classroom instructors/lecturers, and preceptors. Through this two-year, million dollar project, subject matter experts have partnered to develop curricula and train clinical scholars and preceptors in the use of simulation technology to enhance skill-based competencies. Faculty orientation workshops for the use and application of simulation tools will be developed and held at the WELLS Center, and on-line coaching and skill- building workshops will be developed to support the use of various technologies to train educators and clinical staff. In addition, the Departments e–Colorado workforce learning management system portal will become the repository for a statewide and/or national virtual mentor clearinghouse for faculty development support.

The aforementioned approaches to the healthcare crisis are examples the State Workforce Development System has developed in response to President Bush's call for innovative workforce solutions built and sustained through strategic partnerships. Critical to all our efforts are the public/ private collaborative partnerships. Though they present unprecedented challenges for government and its processes, these unique initiatives afford us the opportunity to confront the status quo and build for the future.

———

Mrs. MUSGRAVE. Our last witness is Ms. Kay Norton. I would just like to say, President Norton, I very much appreciate you coming to Washington, D.C., and I look forward to working with you on issues for the University. I know you have a number of things to deal with, but this one today is critically important for our quality of life. And with the growth in Colorado, it sounds very similar to the growth in Nevada, Jon, very similar. And demographics being what they are, and of course, in the fourth district of Colorado, I serve a vast rural area. Seventy-five percent of the population is up in Weld and Larimer Counties and Boulder County, but 75 percent of the land mass is out there in those remote rural areas, so some very unique challenges that we're facing here in Colorado.

Ms. Norton has an undergraduate degree in English and a juris doctorate from the University of Denver, College of Law. She joined the University staff in 1998 as Vice-President for University Affairs, General Counsel, and Secretary to the Board of Trustees.

During her tenure at UNC, she has created opportunities to enhance the public health training and service in Colorado. Through the Colorado School of Public Health for Rural, Native American, Hispanic and Inner-City Populations. We're looking forward to your testimony.

STATEMENT OF KAY NORTON, PRESIDENT, UNIVERSITY OF NORTHERN COLORADO, GREELEY, CO

Ms. NORTON. Thank you very much, Congresswoman Musgrave. And it is a privilege to be here with you and with Mr. Porter, and I appreciate the opportunity.

I was at a meeting this morning when I heard for the umteenth time a reference to a very popular book by Thomas Friedman called "The World is Flat," which is about the fact that we are in a global economy, and that from the perspective of a higher education institution, we have to prepare our students for competition on a global basis. And the issue of the preparation of nurses and the shortage of nursing professionals is a worldwide issue. But we can no longer solve that by stealing from each other, or even by recruiting from the Philippines, which has certainly occurred in this country.

So I'm pleased to be able to participate in talking with you today about some of the things that we are doing locally in Colorado, regionally in the western United States, and nationally to address this critical issue.

Most of the statistics have already been mentioned, and there are also some contained in my written testimony, which you have in the record. I would note something that hasn't been mentioned that only 1 percent of the nursing professionals in the State of Colorado have a Ph.D., which is the entry degree required for full faculty status at a university. I appreciate very much Ms. Carparelli's remarks about the importance of higher education institution-based preparation of nursing professionals as we go forward, although the clinical piece is vitally important. On-the-job-training is not enough to really advance the profession and its role in our health care system in the United States.

The University of Northern Colorado School of Nursing is a microcosm of the issue about faculty retirements. One-third of our doctorally prepared nursing faculty retired in 2004 and 2005. And, in fact, our current codirector of our nursing program, we literally talked out of retirement to come back and provide that leadership for us because we knew where she lived. So, she could not escape completely.

But it's an issue that we have already seen played out here on our campus. And it was mentioned that one of the major issues that universities and colleges and community colleges face is that the market has not served us well in terms of the salaries that we are able to pay to faculty. They aren't appropriate for the responsibility and the learning that's required, and we have an issue, as well, in terms of price sensitivity in terms of tuition that we should charge for a professional preparation program for nurses.

Some programs, you can have differential tuition because the market will bear it. Let's say in a business program or particularly at the graduate level. But when you're talking about a public service profession like teaching or like nursing, it's a different question as to how much should you put on the student in order to bear the cost of paying faculty appropriately. It's something with which we've wrestled, and we need to take a good hard look at that in terms of what the role of state and the Federal Government might be in helping us to perhaps shape the market forces, to make the adjustments that are going to be necessary for us to compensate these professionals appropriately.

I would like to talk to you a bit today about what the University of Northern Colorado has done to respond to the nursing faculty shortage. Most prominently, we started 2 years ago an on-line Ph.D. Program in nursing education. This is not the same sort of

Ph.D. That one would acquire at the University of Colorado Health Sciences Center, for example, where a nursing Ph.D. Is in clinical practice areas and research, as opposed to education. The University of Northern Colorado, as many of you know, began as a teacher preparation institution, a normal school in 1889. It is still by law the center of our reason for being and our public mission is the preparation of education professionals, and particularly at the graduate level.

The program, as I mentioned, was launched in 2004 and it's committed to increasing the number of doctorally prepared nurse educators. Graduates of the Ph.D. Program are qualified, therefore, to fill nursing faculty positions in educational institutions and in health care agencies. It was mentioned, also, that the clinical settings in which nurses are employed also have a significant education and continuing education activity and role in our health care system. Therefore, the graduates of our program are prepared to meet those different types of needs.

The program is delivered on line. We admitted 18 students in the '04-'05 "cohort" we call it, a group that goes through together. Another 18 were admitted in '05-'06.

We're excited about those possibilities and are looking forward to the work that those students are going to be contributing to the research base her and nationally.

We are also proposing that the University of Northern Colorado be the home for a national center for nursing education. We have a similar concept in place here at the University of Northern Colorado that—called the National Center for Low Incidence Disabilities, which addresses another critical need for the education of educators for the blind and the deaf. And that center, as the Center for Nursing Education would do, uses technology to research and develop best practices for providing that type of education and disseminating that information, again, using technology.

Our proposal for the National Center for Nursing Education is in collaboration with the Colorado Center for Nursing Excellence, which has been mentioned a number of times. The National Council of State Boards of Nursing and other state college and university degree programs in nursing, and it has three purposes: To provide academic programs in nursing education, master's and post-master's certificates, Ph.D. Through course offerings on campus, on line, and at outreach sites. Potential outreach sites include locations in the northern, the southern, and the western slope regions of this state, especially in rural and underserved areas that have community colleges that operate associate degree programs in nursing.

Our community colleges and 4 year schools in these areas have attempted to expand their nursing programs, but have the problems that have been described in terms of qualified faculty to staff those programs.

Second, the center would provide professional development opportunities for nurse educators who are in place through summer institutes, teleconferences, webcasts, and on-line educational programs.

And last, we want to establish a national nursing education resource center. Ms. Carparelli mentioned this. That would enable nursing faculty to access information and resources pertaining to contemporary issues and trends in nursing education through a centralized data base, and create a center for evidence-based nursing education; that is research into what works, that will provide faculty and graduate students opportunities to work together in advancing and addressing the question of what should nursing education be. Not only what is it now and what are the current best practices, but how should it fit into the healthcare system as it's developing given that not only the demographics are changing, but the demands and the type of care and the role of the nurse in the continuum from physicians down through what used to be called orderlies, really needs to be addressed. And we are eager to participate and thinking very hard about, well, what should—not only what should a nurse be and how should he or she be prepared, but, you know, how do we accomplish that?

The University has also been partners in developing a multistate consortium that's called NEXUS, N-E-X-U-S. It includes the University of Colorado, the University of Arizona, the University of Utah, and Oregon Health Sciences University to develop a mechanism for students to access Ph.D. Courses on line through a collaborative arrangement.

This is really a sophisticated form of outsourcing, if you will. These courses exist. One of these institutions in the consortium will have the course material and the means for delivering it. It makes no sense to reinvent the wheel and have each state or institution do that work, so we're very excited about that.

Our other efforts are listed in my written testimony, so I will stop here. I do notice, Congressman Porter, that Nevada—there is no Nevada institution listed as a consortium in NEXUS, but perhaps there should be.

Mr. PORTER. I agree.

Mrs. MUSGRAVE. Thank you very much for your testimony.

[The prepared statement of Ms. Norton follows:]

Statement of Kay Norton, President, University of Northern Colorado, Greeley, CO

The Nursing Faculty Shortage

By the year 2020 the U.S. Bureau of Labor (2003) projects that there will be a shortfall of 800,000 nurses. The shortage is more acute in rural areas as it is more difficult for rural health care providers to recruit qualified nursing staff; rural health care facilities take 60% longer than urban facilities to fill nursing vacancies [1]; almost half of frontier nurses have the ADN as their highest degree compared to non-frontier nurses. Although enrollment in entry-level baccalaureate programs in nursing increased 10.6% in 2004 over the previous year, nursing colleges and universities denied 26,340 qualified applications due primarily to a shortage of nurse educators (American Association of Colleges of Nursing, 2004).

The Colorado Center for Nursing Excellence Report, "The 2004 Colorado Nursing Faculty Supply and Demand Study" outlines a critical problem. While enrollment in nursing schools has increased in recent years, it is stalling now at a critical juncture, because there are not enough faculty to handle the workload. Colorado's shortage of qualified nursing faculty at its two year nursing schools is three times the national average, and nearly double the national average at its four year schools. Only 1% of nursing professionals in the state have a Ph.D.

It is anticipated that the faculty shortage will worsen as the average age of nursing faculty is 53 with increasing numbers of faculty preparing to retire. It is esti-

---

[1] MacPhee, M and Scott, J. (2002) The role of social support networks for rural hospital nurses: Supporting and sustaining the rural nursing work force. Journal of Nursing Administration, 32(5):264–272.

mated that between 200 to 300 doctorally prepared faculty are eligible for retirement from 2003 to 2012. The University of Northern Colorado's School of Nursing is a microcosm of this problem as one-third of the doctorally prepared nursing faculty at UNC retired in 2004 and 2005.

The University of Northern Colorado is taking the lead in addressing the shortage of nurses and nursing educators. UNC prepares master's and doctoral nursing faculty through the delivery of an online Ph.D. program in Nursing Education, the creation of the National Center for Nursing Education, and the master's and baccalaureate degrees in nursing.

The University of Northern Colorado Online Ph.D. Program in Nursing Education

The primary mission of UNC's online Ph.D. in Nursing Education is to establish excellence in nursing education. The doctoral program prepares nurses to contribute to developing leadership in nursing education, the scholarship of teaching, and education based-research in the discipline. The program is committed to increasing the number of doctorally prepared nurse educators. Graduates of the PhD program are qualified to fill nursing faculty positions in educational institutions and health care agencies. The program is delivered online. We admitted 18 students in our first year (04–05) and 18 students in our second year (05–06). The interest in and demand for the program has been overwhelming. Although the program is certainly designed to address the shortage of faculty in the state of Colorado, students from across the country compete for admission to this unique program. Each summer the students from UNC's PhD program come together at the National Nurse Educator Conference of the Rockies where they share the latest in educational research and "best practice" with nurse educators from around the country. Last summer, PhD students were presented with the opportunity to dialogue with Dr. Patricia Benner, nationally known nurse theorist and researcher. Furthermore UNC's PhD students have been participating in collaborative research efforts with the Colorado Center for Nursing Excellence to address nurse recruitment and retention issues in Colorado. The University of Northern Colorado's PhD program and the Colorado Center for Nursing Excellence will partner to conduct research to address future issues of importance to nursing education in Colorado.

We have also been partners in a multi-state consortium, NEXUS, which includes University of Northern Colorado, University of Colorado, University of Arizona, University of Utah, and Oregon Health Sciences University to develop a mechanism for students to access PhD courses on-line through a collaborative arrangement.

The University of Northern Colorado's National Center for Nursing Education

The UNC School of Nursing, in partnership with the Colorado Center for Nursing Excellence, the National Council of State Boards of Nursing, and state associate degree, baccalaureate, and higher degree programs in nursing, is working to develop the National Center for Nursing Education. The Center will have the following three purposes: 1) Provide academic programs in nursing education (master's, post-master's certificate, and PhD) through course offerings on the main campus in Greeley, online, and at outreach sites. Potential outreach sites include locations in the northern, southern, and western-slope regions of the state, especially in rural and underserved areas having community colleges that operate associate degree programs in nursing. 2) Provide professional development opportunities for nurse educators through summer institutes, teleconferences, webcasts, and online educational programs; and 3) Establish a National Nursing Education Resource Center that will a) enable nursing faculty to access information and resources pertaining to contemporary issues and trends in nursing education through a centralized database; and b) create a center for evidence-based nursing education that will provide faculty and graduate students in nursing education with opportunities for multidisciplinary, interdisciplinary, and multi-institutional research in nursing education.

Other University of Northern Colorado Nursing Programs

Online Graduate Program in Nursing Education

UNC's School of Nursing also offers a Graduate Certificate in Nursing Education program online to master's prepared nurses, matriculated master's nursing students, and matriculated doctoral students who wish to augment their professional studies with advanced coursework in nursing education and academic roles. We have 9 new admits in Fall 2005.

Online RN to BSN program

Student demand for easier access to the Bachelor of Science in Nursing program, particularly in rural Colorado, led to the development of the RN to BSN online program in 1998. The RN to BSN program is 2 year online program for individuals who have an Associates Degree in Nursing or a Diploma in nursing. The online RN to BSN program takes 4 semesters to complete, clinical hours are arranged where students are living, and nurses are able to work full-time while completing the program. Students are admitted every Fall. The program has averaged 12 students per cohort. We've received 30 applications for Fall 2005.

Second Degree Accelerated BSN program with local hospitals

The second degree accelerated BSN program is designed to meet the needs of those students who are seeking a BSN as a second bachelor's degree. Admission to the accelerated second degree program is competitive. First priority is given to qualified candidates who are committed to living and working in the Northern Colorado area. All applicants are sponsored by and commit to work for a minimum of two years at Poudre Valley Health System or North Colorado Medical Center/Banner Health upon graduation. This program is privately funded by these two facilities and each system provides financial support to their selected candidates and students complete their applicable clinical courses at the sponsoring facility. Students admitted to the second degree accelerated program will be able to complete the nursing courses in 20 months (vs. 26). The program has been in place since 2002 and we admit approximately 18 students each year.

Summary

The inception of UNC's PhD nursing program has been instrumental in laying the foundation for increasing the number of highly qualified nurse educators. Our participation in the NEXUS partnership reflects the recognition that UNC provides a unique resource in addressing the acute shortage of nurse educators in the region as well as the state. In keeping with UNC's education mission, we have taken the lead in addressing the shortage of doctorally prepared nursing educators and will be a national leader in nursing education with the creation of the National Center for Nursing Education.

———

Mrs. MUSGRAVE. It has been brought to my attention that the service workers' union are out in the foyer and I don't know if they can hear me, but I just want them to know that they can submit written material for the record and I'd be happy to include that in the record today. And if any of the witnesses here will include all of your written material, and if you have any other studies or anything that you would like to submit, we'd be happy to have those.

We'll go ahead and start the questioning now. I think I'll start with you, Sue, if I may. And you talked about not very many men or minorities being attracted to the profession right now. I can imagine that it's a great advantage if a nurse has a second language also, and so there are many benefits for bringing men and minorities into the profession, and I'd just like to know strategies that you have for bringing more in.

Ms. CARPARELLI. The statistics that I quoted to you reflect, I think the patterns, the historical patterns, which certainly, obviously, nursing has been a profession that has attracted many more women than men. What we know is that we are going a better job of recruiting both males and females into the profession, and our schools are becoming more diverse in their enrollment, both by gender as well as by ethnicity.

We have observed some interesting trends in our state, and I would imagine that they would be consistent with other states as well. In relation to the attractiveness of the profession post 9/11, there were several things that happened in our country. We had tremendous job loss, and that job loss, in our state in particular, was experienced by those who were at high educational levels. They were knowledge workers. And the other phenomenon that I observed was that that experience post–9/11 caused us to really reflect purpose and meaning of work and that folks who had previously been employed, for example, in the tech sector, which was very high growth, high paid positions in our state, but perhaps low personal fulfillment.

People who were looking to retool for jobs that were never going to return to our economy looked at jobs that provided more personal fulfillment by virtue of service to others. And I think that that has been benefited us greatly in terms of the numbers of both men and women who have considered these career fields.

I would say to you that we have very important work to do in our K through 12 educational process. If we do not do a good job of science and math, foundational skill building, people who may have aptitude and interest will not be able to be successful in what is a very rigorous academic program.

And our state, as other states, is challenged by that reality and we find ourselves in our schools of nursing, at times, having to do remedial work in order to retain very capable students who come perhaps not with the essential foundational skills that are required, and we find that in particular within our community college programs.

Elise spoke about some of the skill building programs that the Department of Labor has helped to fund and maintains in our state that are essential to that process.

Mrs. MUSGRAVE. How do you think that's being communicated to K–12 educators and administrators?

Ms. CARPARELLI. I think that—I think that K through 12 administrators and teachers do understand that these math and science skills are essential. I think that they don't necessarily connect all the dots in terms of relevancy to the array of career fields that those skills require as foundational. I certainly know that UNC, amongst other of our teacher preparation programs, are working to assist in that effort, and I know that our school districts across the state are looking at curriculum and teaching methodologies that will support student learning in that area.

That said, it's a long path, and one that we must persist in, not just for these health care careers, but for the array of knowledge-based jobs and professions that now are the future of our economy.

Mrs. MUSGRAVE. I appreciate that. Having served on a local board of education, I wish that boards of education around the State of Colorado could hear these remarks today. And one of my goals as a board member was academic rigor. You know, we know that students have—they mature—the maturation levels are very difference, and I would like academic rigor in K–12 so that when they want to make a choice, they then can.

And remedial efforts are very expensive and time consuming, and you know, we would hope that school boards around the Nation would hear these things, because you're talking about the world being flat, the book and the global economy and the academic rigor is so important, again, as you said, not only in this field, but for our students to be ready for that global economy out there. Thank you.

Mr. Porter, do you have questions?

Mr. PORTER. My first question is about getting old.

Mrs. MUSGRAVE. I thought 47 sounded kind of young.

Mr. PORTER. Sue, I appreciate it. But having crossed that half century mark, I think I'm pretty young, but I guess I'm not.

But thank you all for your testimony today. I actually have some questions, and you're all welcome to answer or if you choose not to, that's OK. But I'm trying to compile some data for my own decisionmaking.

Maybe it's in the background, and I read your testimony prior to today, but also was looking and may have missed it. But how many professional instructors do we need? I know we're going to be short by almost 800,000-some health care professionals in the next 10, 15, 20 years, but what should our goal be for the professional in the classroom? What percentage should we be—what should be our goal?

Ms. DIERKER. I'll say while we need we need more, one of the things that the study showed is that really we don't have a very good baseline, we don't have really well-defined data elements and data collection, so that even among educators in programs, there's been so much rapid sort of change and dislocation and numbers and the use of technology and the change from old models of teaching to what we should do with new ways of teaching, using technology, that there are some fundamental questions that we need to really get to in terms of what should education look like to prepare the competent professional for the 21st century. What does that really look like? How do we take advantage of distance learning and all of these other things to sort of say there are numbers, there are ratios of how many we need?

What we do recognize, and this is, again, I'm speaking on behalf of the informants who really brought it forward out of the study, is that we've really got to do some fundamental innovation in what nursing education looks like to go from the old sort of apprentice model to really a really solid professional knowledge worker who has real critical thinking skills that can be applied in diverse and increasingly challenging settings.

And so I think that's where we really need to work with some of the leaders in education and practice to really get at your question, which is "what does the model look like?" and then how would we project and then collect data over some time and really do that in a concerted way with a research agenda that gives us some rapid but sound answers.

Mr. PORTER. What concerns me is we have state-of-the-art operating rooms now across the country, the latest in technology. But it seems to me that some of the training may still be from 50 years ago or 100 years ago, and I want to make sure we know what the goal is. And you say 800,000 professionals, I think there's a weak link and that's something we need to work on is how we can come up with some form of delivery and consistency.

Ms. DIERKER. Well, and I will say in Colorado, and I'm sure this is happening in Nevada, but in states, as everyone's grappling with this, we have some remarkable demonstration projects underway, as you've heard. And I think we need to be listening and talking and learning from them on an ongoing, constant, basis to get at your issue of "what's the model?" and "what should we be striving for?" because those are the laboratories where people are trying to figure it out, and use these technologies and examples from other industries, actually, like the airline industry, where they realize that you get precision and safety when you use simulation and you use certain teaching methods so that pilots don't make mistakes.

And so we have some ways to learn about that. And like I say, in our study, it showed that even in rural areas and—as soon as people are introduced to these technologies and these new teaching methods, there is a hunger for them. We just need to—people want the support and the help to design curriculum and have resources to connect all the dots and have the programmatic sort of institutionalized ways to go at it.

Mr. PORTER. And by the way, and I appreciate the study, I'm sure we could just cross out Colorado and put Nevada and it would be almost identical, so I look forward to using this as a resource, too. Thank you.

Anyone else want to comment?

Ms. NORTON. I might just give you an estimate. If we made no changed in how we educate nurses, and I certainly think we do need to, everything that Lynn has just described, needs to happen. But we do know that 200–300 doctorally prepared faculty will be eligible to retire nationally from 2003 to 2012, and so if we were going to replace them and expand capacity, we'd be looking at needing Ph.D.s in the 100's or low thousands would be a very rough estimate. The number is probably higher than lower——

Mr. PORTER. Excuse me, so what you're saying is that the status quo——

Ms. NORTON. Right.

Mr. PORTER.—we're going to lose 300.

Ms. NORTON. Right.

Mr. PORTER. And even with status quo, it's really not enough.

Ms. NORTON. And that—and status quo hasn't allowed us to expand programs to meet the need for the 800,000——

Mr. PORTER. Because we're already short 800,000——

Ms. NORTON. Correct.

Mr. PORTER.—or whatever it is.

Ms. NORTON. Correct.

Mr. PORTER. So you think in the thousands.

Ms. NORTON. Yeah, in the low thousands, right. Four figures.

Mr. PORTER. Thank you. And I know it was mentioned earlier about the book, "The World is Flat," and I'd like to reference—if I could write a book, and I'm not a very good writer, it would be about the world as we know it, even here inside of the boundaries of the U.S. I have found that, when it comes to education, whether it be higher education, health care profession, or even primary and secondary, we have created these paradigms and these little worlds and each one has their own thing. You've got the school district doing their own thing, you've got the universities doing their own thing, you've got local governments doing their own thing, you've got private sector doing their own thing. And the world really is flat right here in Colorado and Nevada and Iowa where I grew up. We have everyone in their little worlds, and I think it's time that, as mentioned in the collaborative effort, I think it was mentioned here numerous times, that it's the responsibility for health care for local government also. It's a responsibility for the legislature. Of course, they know that they have a role. But we have created little worlds and little boxes and we're not crossing over, and I think that we need to do a cultural change ourselves as policymakers and leaders that health care is as important to the local government as it is to the University of Northern Colorado or CU, which we were talking about earlier. I hear a lot about CU from my chief of staff, but I am very concerned that we also have this paradigm when it comes to retired professionals.

I know Nevada is fastest growing in retirees. Well, there's a wealth of talent in our retiree health care professionals, and as I mention that, I guess I'd like to know, is there a program in place to help bring those retirees back into educational processes and use them in a clinical setting to help train nurses? Is there something in place in Colorado for the retirees?

Ms. CARPARELLI. OK, since I'm the one that raised the age issues, I'll tackle that one. And let me just respond to that first by saying that age is important in these very physically demanding jobs. That we know that, for example, in an acute care environment, that the physical rigor of being a staff nurse, a direct care provider, makes it difficult for people to perform in that role much past mid-50's because of the demands of that job. And so,——

Mr. PORTER. If I may interrupt, what would the average tenure be, then, of someone to retire in their mid-50's? How long would they have been in the profession? Is that 30 years, 20 years, 10 years.

Ms. CARPARELLI. Well, it would obviously depend when they entered into the profession, and we have many nurses who began their educational process right out of high school and have been practicing in that profession since that time.

Increasingly, as you look at the age of our students currently enrolled, we are seeing a much older student population, particularly in our community colleges and our accelerated nursing programs. We are seeing people retooling, as I spoke about before, from other professions to prepare for a new career path within nursing. And so they are in their late 20's to early 30's as they are starting this profession.

Mr. PORTER. Is it as much age as it is the length of time in the profession? Is there just a burnout happening after so many years or is it a combination of age and just worn out from the profession.

Ms. CARPARELLI. I think there are a variety of factors. I think that the work environment has many elements that create burnout and dissatisfaction for those who work within that environment. I think that the increased level of acuity within our—patient acuity within the acute care environment means that people are sicker and they stay a very short period of time, and so it makes for a very intense work experience with little time for the satisfiers that those within this profession are looking for in terms of a relationship with that patient.

I think that there are also substantial cost pressures that providers struggle with that create productivity pressures upon individual care providers that in turn create dissatisfaction on the part of those that are in direct care delivery modes.

I think that there are a whole host of issues that need to be addressed in effort to retain health care providers, nurses, amongst them.

We do know that we have to make some modifications in the process of work, and we have a variety of initiatives that reflect that. If you've not heard about efforts, particularly on the part of acute care environments to create magnate status, which is an element that focuses on the work environment for the professional practice of nursing, and we don't have necessarily time to get into that, but it is an example of efforts being undertaken to substantially modify and make more satisfying and more rewarding the professional practice of nursing within the care delivery system.

That said, as is the case with K through 12 education, we have a great deal of work to be done in that regard, and it is essential that nurses, as participants in that process, have substantial input and say as to how that works for them. Their voice in this process is essential.

There is opportunity for us with the aging; particularly of the clinical experts to be able to bring them into teaching roles. What we know is that it is imperative that those——

Mr. PORTER. Excuse me, when you say—so I understand—clinical expert" is someone that has field training is now in the training position? Is that the term you use for teachers.

Ms. CARPARELLI. A clinical expert is someone who has clinical expertise—current knowledge and practice within a particular area of practice. As an example,——

Mr. PORTER. And those are more apt to be the—those individuals would be the instructors.

Ms. CARPARELLI. Those are the people, for example, who may have 20 years of experience in labor and delivery, 30 years of experience in labor delivery, and either are looking for a means to augment their practice by adding a teaching component to that, or are looking for a way to move into a next stage of a professional career.

My point is that what we are finding is that these people whose job it is to provide care, and who are experts in the delivery of certain kinds of care, are able and willing to participate as clinical instructors, teaching students those clinical skills in partnership with their educational institutions when supported through some basic orientation, training, mentoring, and coaching around how to teach.

Now, that said, they will not nor should they ever substitute for the kind of folks that President Norton is speaking about as it relates to faculty, but they can augment and support the learning and bring to the student experience great expertise and experience in certain kinds of clinical areas.

So it's an example of the kind of collaboration between practice and education that can happen and must happen to create the kind of quality learning experiences that students need.

Mr. PORTER. I have more questions, but I'll wait if that's OK.

Mrs. MUSGRAVE. OK, I'll bring some forth. Could you comment on technology, whichever one wants to, particularly simulation? I don't know who wants to take that.

Ms. DIERKER. Certainly in the study, we asked our informants to what degree they were already starting to and were interested in using technology so that I can comment to some degree on what came out of the study and some of what I know otherwise just by way of background.

But the kinds of technologies that are really emerging now include some of the things that President Norton mentioned, which are ways of education that rely on on-line curriculum and sort of didactic methods. But in the clinical setting, there are simulation technologies that are partially self-directed on-line methods, but also involve literally mannequins and lifelike—very life-like mannequins who can provide a kind of experience much like, again, to use the airline example, of being in a cockpit where you really have a patient and you can simulate situations of physical crisis, birth, certain kinds of physical—physiologic states, and students and teams of students can literally practice taking care of a patient in that environment.

And so that what you have, then, is a way for an instructor—for people to not only watch and observe, like the old days when I went to nursing school, and you might crowd around a bed and get to actually see someone in a certain state. And this way, with simulation, you really have students who can go through the entire continuum of how you'd care for that patient, have instruction, repeat it, practice it, and get it right.

And so these are the kinds of technologies that both hospitals and schools are putting into place and that they are referring to when they talk about trying to rely on technology.

What the study found is that while you can buy a mannequin and you can put it there and say, "OK, here we have it," there's a lot—there's a big gap between that and having faculty who know how to teach using it and really know how to integrate a student who has come in with computer-based background and the simulation technology and integrate all of that into a valuable learning experience. And that's where faculty needs support.

Mrs. MUSGRAVE. That's what I was really hoping to understand. You know, I see how it could very much improve the quality of the education, but what I don't understand is how it really addresses the shortage of faculty, you know. I know that instructors can use that, but you still have to have the instructors, I would imagine, the teachers there. So, I don't know if you want to comment further on that or not.

Ms. CARPARELLI. I'd like to comment on that. Your point is exactly right on. The use of these emerging technologies does not take the place of the instructor nor does it take the place of learning that takes place in the clinical environment. But what it can do is to augment the student learning or to rehearse, essentially, things that the student will see in the clinical environment in preparation for that clinical experience.

And I think the important point is that faculty need time and support to be able to, themselves, learn how to use these emerging technologies effectively and they need time to conduct the research to determine efficacy relative to learning and outcomes.

And, again, it's part of what President Norton referred to in terms of evidence-based education. We need to learn how to use this stuff effectively, and we're in many instances at the front end in the use of this technology and the faculty experts haven't yet had the opportunity to test it and evaluate it and research it in the ways that we have more historically teaching methodology.

So that becomes a very important aspect of what needs to happen as it relates to education.

Ms. NORTON. If I may add, four of doctoral students in our nursing education Ph.D. Program are focusing on the use of simulation technology and nursing education right now.

Ms. DIERKER. And I just wanted to, again, make a point about, I think your issue about how does this really contribute to supply and where we're going to get it. I think one of the things that we revealed, which was pretty stunning in our study, when we asked representatives from the hospitals and long-term care facilities, you know, "how much money are you really spending on nursing education?" And we got a large number. I mean, when you think of $2 million in a year from the people we surveyed who, you know, they range, of course, some of the big systems with the larger numbers, but still, that's a lot where they're literally putting up money to backfill, to support the need for further education and strengthening of those students.

So to your question, Mr. Porter, about how many do we need, when and where? We've got to incorporate these sort of methods to sort of answer that question, because out there in the practicing world, you have these hospital systems that have a large component of their budget going to staff that need to cover their new grads just because they can't practice independently, full practice yet, and need to train students.

And so how many of them do we need, how many could we free up? How much do we take a financial burden off of the industry? That, of course, cycles back into costs and cycles around to what we all pay.

So, I mean, they're all interrelated, which is why we're got to figure an efficiency equation about how we can best educated people.

Mrs. MUSGRAVE. I was interested, President Norton, when you talked about the difference between 2 year schools and 4 year schools and the shortage of faculty. Could you address that, please.

Ms. NORTON. Yes. Well, there are different levels of preparation of nursing professionals because a nurse is not necessarily a nurse is a nurse. You have the traditional licensure frame of references, LPN, more like a 2-year program; BSN—RN, more like a bachelor's program, although they're not the same thing. This is all something that I had to learn a lot about as we addressed the issue here at the University.

And the 2 year programs produce an AND nurse, who is certainly fully prepared to do many functions in an acute care facility and in long-term care facilities, but would not necessarily be prepared, for example, to do work in the surgical units or other more sophisticated areas.

And so as we look at need, we have to look at what sort of nurse do we need where and how many and at what level can we adequately prepare those students. So the answer is not simply to say, "Well, let's just have everybody do a 2-year program," because that won't necessarily be the right level of preparation for where the need is.

So it's another mismatch in this rather complicated picture that we have to take a look at. And if I may, I'd like to just mention in terms of the issue about technology and how does it help. Our experience in higher education has been that technology tends not to save money so much as it enables us to increase quality and, very importantly, increase access and the dissemination of information. But it adds sophistication and it can contribute to quality and it can certainly cost a lot of money, but it doesn't necessarily eliminate the need for human beings and those knowledge workers.

Mrs. MUSGRAVE. Mr. Porter.

Mr. PORTER. You're going to be sorry you invited me today, but I'm——

Mrs. MUSGRAVE. Good thing we don't have the light.

Mr. PORTER. It's probably a good thing. I would be in trouble. In my approach to public services, I am not an expert; you're the expert, so I try to learn as much as I can from you. I'd rather hear from you than you hear from me.

But there is a few things. Average tenure; what is it for a professional? How long do they stay in the profession? Is it—I know we started to go down that path; is it 10 years, 20 years, 15? I know there's lots of variables, but how long would they stay?

Ms. CARPARELLI. Are you talking about practicing?

Mr. PORTER. Practicing.

Ms. CARPARELLI. Practicing nurses, I think it's extremely variable, and I think that we can learn a lot by looking at that variability. We have a high rate of attrition from the profession in the first three to 5 years out of school. And that has to do, again, with a variety of factors, but it's an important consideration because we do not get the full benefit of all of those that we educated.

Mr. PORTER. As part of that, leaving a family or relocation or spouse's relocation, or some of those things.

Ms. CARPARELLI. As I said, there are a variety of factors. Some leave because it wasn't what they expected——

Mr. PORTER. Absolutely.

Ms. CARPARELLI.—and they do not find it be a satisfying work environment, they don't find——

Mr. PORTER. But is it higher in nursing than in other industries.

Ms. CARPARELLI. I would not feel qualified to fully answer that question. I think it would be important to, you know, perhaps think about who you wanted to compare that to.

Mr. PORTER. Yeah.

Ms. CARPARELLI. I think——

Mr. PORTER. So we don't—and I hate to interrupt, because I know we're running a little low on time, but so right now we'd say we really don't know an average tenure, right? Is that what I'm hearing? That's something we'd probably need to find out.

Employer. Who is the largest employer? Is it the hospitals?

Ms. CARPARELLI. Yes.

Mr. PORTER. That's the largest. And I'll be honest with you, I don't have a lot of sympathy for the private sector when it comes to training. I think they share a huge responsibility. I don't think this is just a public sector responsibility to train and to recruit and encourage health care professionals. I think industry should be the leader in helping find not only the nurses, but the clinical instructor. They should play a bigger role in all of this, so I don't have a lot of sympathy in that they've made an investment. That's their responsibility also, because the Federal Government, the state and local governments, even though health care is a quality of life issue, I think the hospitals need to do more, and I've heard even the hospitals in Nevada talk about the trouble they're having getting qualified and trained professionals, and well, if you compare nursing to other areas in the private sector, the private sector steps up and trains people to fit into their profession, whether it be at Southwest Airlines, Microsoft, or a Ma & Pa restaurant, they train and they feel that they want to have the best and the brightest working for them.

So I guess one thing, and I know that I'm going to carry forward with my colleague, is finding ways—where the barriers are to the private sector. I'm sure there's lots of reasons, from the costs and there may be more incentives, but they need to step up to the plate and help us more than they are, and this is something that I plan on working with, and I'd say in a proactive way. I'm not into mandates and penalizing, but we need to find out from the professional—the hospitals what we can do to help them get more involved, because they're hands on and they need to have some training—more training internally.

Ms. LOWE-VAUGHN. Representative Porter, one of the things that's so exciting about the partnerships in Colorado is this very issue. Our partners from the private sector, the hospitals, the acute care, the long-term care, all of these partners, including education, have stepped forward and have put together four-to-one matches on all of the grants that we've been doing. They're working with all of our local workforce regions and private regional collaboratives to improve the nursing population and allied health care. So I think Colorado is a model for those kind of collaborative partnerships, and we're very pleased that industry has come to the table and talked to us about the very issues which started the dialog here.

Mr. PORTER. And I appreciate that, but I think that the private sector can do more.

Ms. LOWE-VAUGHN. Sure.

Mr. PORTER. And when I talk about the flat world we live in, I'm including the private sector because I do hear from private sector, not only in Nevada, but across the country, and their resistance to being more involved in training that they want someone else to do more. So I applaud those here in Colorado, and I'm sure that it's probably even unique. But I think we can do more, and we can encourage more of that.

A question, and again, the study is great, and I've just had a chance to leaf through it and you've spent some time, you know, talking about what the clinical professional makes in the rural and urban areas, but if we could just summarize real briefly. If you were to take a practicing registered nurse, where they would max out in a salary, if we look at a career path, where they would max out as opposed to a trainer or a teacher or a clinical professional? How do they compare; the practicing nurse to the professional? And you may have touched upon it earlier, but I missed it.

Ms. DIERKER. Well, we didn't do a great deal on the study because of the time and the way in which we went about it given the issues at hand. But, I would say that especially with the competitiveness for a nurse in the hospital setting now, where salaries and bonuses for nurses to be employed in certain settings have really bumped up the clinical range. I think, you know, I'm going to ballpark, because we don't have a lot to go there, but I would say even starting, you know, you're going to end up with a differential of maybe, you know, it depends where you are, of course, but even $10,000. And so then it just sort of widens and it depends on your experience and——

Mr. PORTER. So $10,000 more to be an instructor.

Ms. DIERKER. Clinical—in a clinical—less to be an instructor. Less. I mean, we came up with an average salary for an entry-level faculty of $39,000. Well, you can go in as——

Mr. PORTER. Well, that's a serious problem.

Ms. DIERKER. That's a serious problem.

Mr. PORTER. When you look at a career path.

Ms. DIERKER. And it's worse in rural areas.

Ms. NORTON. The gap is really more like $20,000.

Ms. DIERKER. Right.

Ms. NORTON. At least.

Mr. PORTER. How are they, then, compared to other—let me use the word teacher.

Ms. NORTON. Right.

Mr. PORTER. That's easier for me. For the teacher compared to another field of study, how are they paid; is it similar.

Ms. NORTON. Our faculty salaries in nursing are at the midrange of our faculty salaries,——

Mr. PORTER. They top out at the mid-range.

Ms. NORTON.—generally based on market, and that's why I say the market has failed us somewhat in not really recognizing a shortage, and I think it will adjust. But, for example, a business faculty, the highest paid professors that you'll find on a campus or faculty in a medical school or a law school, the professional—and engineers are also—engineering faculty are in very short supply and command high salaries, often approaching or into the six figures. And your nursing professional faculty, education faculty, are going to be somewhat below that.

Mr. PORTER. So from a career path——

Ms. NORTON. Yeah.

Mr. PORTER.—it's difficult for someone to maybe go backwards.

Ms. NORTON. Exactly. That's the issue. That is absolutely the issue is our faculty may decide that they want to retire because they can make $20,000 or $30,000 a year more going back into clinical practice. And so how do we deal with that gap is an immediate issue that we have to figure out how we deal with.

Mr. PORTER. Again, looking at—the reason we're here, of course, is pretty broad, but specifically to the nursing faculty, you know, there's recruiting problems for new nurses, I mean, there's four or five keys, but when we get down to a career path——

Ms. NORTON. Right.

Mr. PORTER.—why would someone want to leave—unless they were just burnt out and wanted to move on in their profession, why would they want to become a faculty member.

Ms. NORTON. And I think it's also the job satisfaction and really the passion issue that Sue Carparelli mentioned. And maybe they just don't know any better, I don't know.

Mr. PORTER. And don't get me wrong, I applaud everyone for that.

Ms. NORTON. It is a matter of finding that kind of satisfaction, but obviously there's no—we have a huge hurdle in terms of convincing individuals that they want to be nursing faculty, although we turned away students for our Ph.D. Program because of lack of capacity. There's only so much pin-up demand. I mean, the real issue is how do we get some of these younger folks, when you look at the numbers of how many—how few practitioners in nursing generally are under the age of 30. It's striking. Therefore, how many——

Mr. PORTER. Excuse me, if I can interrupt. I think whatever the business profession, people like to have kind of a path and I have spent the bulk of my time in public service with primary and secondary education, so I know more about it, and I see a lot of great classroom teachers that max out that have to become principals and administrators just—not because they really want to do that, but they have to for their career path to support their family.

So I guess the one thing I'm hearing consistently this morning and in fairness I applaud those folks that go to the faculty, but we need to find a way to elevate that position to help as part of a full career path to keep these young folks, when they shoot down the road, that there are some things that they could look forward to because we need those professionals to go—to become faculty. And it's very difficult, I would think, to make that jump.

Ms. NORTON. It is, and it's very challenging and we have to figure out how do we assist the market in figuring that out. I mean, certainly we're willing to do our part. I certainly understand, as an administrator of a university, that we're going to have to figure out how we make those adjustments and really respond as a market generally would respond to the fact that this is a shortage and we have to make it attractive.

And I think you've also mentioned an issue that we see every day in the nursing profession and the teaching profession is the people going into leadership positions not because they want to be leaders, but because of the financial goals that—and needs that they may have and the creation of true leaders in these professions is also crucial. Leaders and educators.

Mrs. MUSGRAVE. It's kind of bewildering to me that this lag time in the market is—I don't know, this seems like an exceptionally long lag time, because we're all seen this coming. You know, we've been talking about it for years, we know what the demographics are, and so this, you know, trying to ascertain why the market has not responded more quicker, is kind of bewildering to me.

Ms. DIERKER. Well, I think one of the things I certainly heard in the study is the sense that our constraints on higher education in our state, in our fiscal situation related to higher ed, has made it difficult for schools to respond by bumping up the salaries. So, because most of our nursing programs are publicly funded here, we don't have a lot of private, so that's been a big issue. It's a convergence of factors that have really been especially difficult.

Mrs. MUSGRAVE. You know, I don't know too many people that want to move forward in a career and take less money.

Mr. PORTER. Well, this is politics, Marilyn.

Mrs. MUSGRAVE. Well, you have a bigger title.

Mr. PORTER. No, that's a choice.

Mrs. MUSGRAVE. You begged for the job, you know.

Mr. PORTER. That's true.

Mrs. MUSGRAVE. Well, I thank you for your testimony today. It has been just extraordinary, and I know that the Congressman and I both would like to do more with this issue and we expect, President Norton, that you will let us know how we can do that. Again, the quality of life issue is out there for the entire United States, but it seems that some areas have even more severe shortages than others, and we need to address that.

Congressman Porter, do you have any final remarks you'd like to make?

Mr. PORTER. Well, I could talk for hours, so I won't. I just appreciate your insights, your comments, your research, because if you don't tell us, as Members of Congress, we don't know. You know, we deal with thousands of issues every day, and I think we're ADD to be Members of Congress, because there are so many issues. But I firmly believe there's not an issue more important to the future of our country than our health care. And there's no one that's more important than the nursing professionals—the professionals in health care delivery, and I get the terms wrong, but those folks out there that are on the front line, the professionals, and we need to find a way to elevate this profession and encourage our young folks and those who want a career change to get into the field.

But I firmly believe there's not a more important issue for us as a country than to focus on getting folks into this field. We can't afford to have the attrition. We can't afford to allow the rest of the world to move in front of us. But more importantly, we need to make sure that, as Members of Congress, we're able to give you the tools you need to get the job done, and that's why I really appreciate being here, I appreciate your insights, and we'll take what I've learned today and move forward. And you will be hearing from me more in the future. So thank you all very, very much. I appreciate it.

And to—we brought staff here from D.C., thank you.

Mrs. MUSGRAVE. Yes.

Mr. PORTER. There's two that came from D.C. I'd like to thank our Committee staff for being here today also. Thank you.

Mrs. MUSGRAVE. I, too, appreciate the staff and their work very much. All of those issues that we deal with as Members of Congress, we are very much assisted by our staff and we appreciate them so very much. I have one of mine traveling with me today, Nina, so Amanda and Nina and whoever else helped out, we appreciate it so very much.

I think it's somewhat paradoxical that when we talk about these shortages of faculty training the nurses, and we hope more and more will come into the profession, men and minorities joining, women, I believe the expectations of patients are even higher and higher. So we really have an interesting dilemma here. We expect quality, excellent health care. And thank goodness there are folks that want to get into the profession and those that want to teach, so we can have that quality of health care.

Thank you very much.

Mr. PORTER. Excuse me, Marilyn, can I add one more thing?

Mrs. MUSGRAVE. Certainly.

Mr. PORTER. It's important to note that I think we're in our infancy and I think now is the time. Even with my concerns, I think we're in our infancy in the future of health care, and that's why what we're talking about today I think can make such a difference in the future, because what's around the corner with technology, and you've talked about it this morning, and what's around the corner in health care, and I just want to again to reiterate my optimism that this is a field that's changing with a lot of complex issues, but you get along very well. We deal with issues where it's divide and conquer, because there are so many folks on issues that hate each other. But what's great about this issue is there is a spirit of cooperation. And I know that we have our—you know, we hang our laundry out in different places, and maybe there are times that we don't agree, but that's another reason why I'm so optimistic about my—what I believe as the challenges for health care, because of the cooperation. It's really refreshing that this industry, even with its differences and its competing partners, it really works well together. So I wanted to really conclude with saying I think we have a lot of work to do, but we're in our infancy and a lot of good things can happen.

Thank you. I promise I'm finished.

Mrs. MUSGRAVE. We appreciate your comments very much. Thank you for coming to this hearing today, and we appreciate everyone being here.

The meeting is adjourned.

[Whereupon, at 11:45 a.m., the Subcommittee was adjourned.]

○

APEX
TP_CF
9780160765193

76523826 — 42